THE UNKNOWN ABOUT THE HUMAN AURA
The Human Aura from a Medical Point of View

THE UNKNOWN ABOUT THE HUMAN AURA

The Human Aura from a Medical Point of View

By

NAWAR SABAH AJWAD

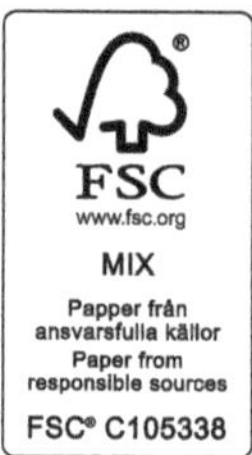©Nawar Sabah Ajwad 2018

Published by: BoD – Books on Demand, Stockholm, Sweden

Printed by: BoD – Books on Demand, Norderstedt, Germany

ISBN: 978-91-7785-387-9

"The mere looking at externals is a matter for clowns, but the intuition of internals is a secret which belongs to physicians"
Paracelsus

Introduction

Since ancient times man has always tried to understand the unusual
and the ambiguous phenomena that occur to him. People
sometimes become sick or well for no reasonable or obvious
reasons. People used to call these phenomena, supernatural,
because they lack a satisfying medical explanation that explains such
phenomena. People sometimes ignore them and sometimes they
wonder why and how these phenomena occur. By definition, if the
supernatural phenomenon has a medical explanation then it loses its
name as a supernatural and it becomes an ordinary one.
The human body is a complicated functional and constructional unit
that exists during the whole human life.
Medicine in ancient times was too primitive to be able to give
correct answers for many medical problems. It could not
comprehend how the body works perfectly as a whole and complete
unit. In the present time we understand, for example, that insulin

deficiency in the human body causes diabetes and the blockage of the small arteries that nourish the heart muscle causes angina pectoris (pain in the heart muscle) or even a heart attack. Despite this advancement in modern medicine, it did not give the seekers satisfying answers for many manifestations of the phenomena that are related to the human aura and which should be mentioned in the discussion of the health issues of the human body.

Chine's medicine, for example, is one of the attempts that made an approach in this subject. This approach is mostly for the first field of the aura, the etheric body, that envelops and permeates through the whole human body. The chine's medicine attempt is through acupuncture, its related meridians and acupoints.

Shamans used to travel to other "worlds" seeking for answers to cure a sick person or to cure themselves. They sometimes use fire, fresh eggs, oils, special voices, parts of leafy tress and other items. Their methods sometimes have good results without knowing the logical and scientific reasons behind the success in their treatment methods.

Nature has its hidden secrets that we should have enough patience to learn them at a satisfying level of understanding for us who seek the truth behind many natural phenomena.

We as human beings are part of the whole universe and everything that changes in the universe affect us in some way or another.

We people also affect each other in an unconscious way. The human aura is also involved here in what is called the collective unconsciousness that I shall discuss later on.

Every time we think, feel or do things, the human aura changes and affect other human aura of the person or persons nearby in a constructive or destructive way.

During the evolution of human beings on earth, his senses were developed. The whole biological system developed together with the development of the aura that envelops and permeates each part of the human body. The purpose of that developing of the aura is to adapt, likewise the biological system, to various challenging environmental factors on earth. The aura indeed tries to keep the body isolated from the hostile influences of the environment.

When we stop facing challenging in our environment we stop developing our abilities that are saved in our DNA (deoxyribo nucleic acid) and chromosomes as codes. We know now for fact that each group of DNA codes make a single gen that is responsible for a specific ability or character in the human body like seeing, hearing, touching, our types of memory, our eyes color, etc. and amazingly, each sense reflects itself continuously in the aura.

As medicine becomes more advanced as it is in recent time, we begin to understand the mechanism that lies behind different phenomena that used to be called mysterious, ambiguous or supernatural.

This is not a diagnostic or a treatment book but it is an attempt to understand the true relationship between the human aura and the orthodox medicine.

In the following pages I will try to give a general ide about the nature of the human aura with its ambiguous and mystical features and a general ide about the biological system of the human body which is in a close relationship to the human aura as a whole functional and constructional unit of both the human body and its inseparable aura.

Contents

WHAT IS AURA

This book discusses the human aura, therefore we should first take a look at what aura is for something in general, how it looks like, what are its characteristic features, what are the fields that it consists of and the classification of it.

After we have understood part one of this book, it will be easy to understand the rest of the book. Despite that I can describe this book as an organized and valuable source of information that can be read from everywhere in each part, depending on what the reader has for background regarding the subject and its hidden and the unknown secrets that is not available for anyone and it should be available for those who seek the truth behind every scene of event in this amazing subject.

The aura or the subtle body of man is the field of fine biological energy that envelops and permeates through our physical human bodies. Like everything in the universe that can be divided into two parts until infinity times of divisions, the aura consists existentially of many different fields that have different and sometimes arguable names. The arguable names are concerning the fields which are beyond the third field as we will see later on.

Auric fields are mixed with each other in different degrees depending on the type of the field that we deal with.

Most of the schools that describe the aura mention only three fields of the aura, the etheric body, the astral body and the mental body (the word "body" here means the field) for the reason that these fields are the major fields in the aura and they are the major fields that are worthy to mention in the process of treatment of the unhealthy aura.

The real classification of the aura or auric field is indeed beyond this simplicity. We can mention one type of classification which is in a simple way as following: The etheric body, the astral body, the mental body, the causal body, the buddhic body and the atmic body. There are also subdivisions of some of these fields or bodies that are not concerned enough in the auric healthy issues.

There are indeed different schools regarding the classification of the aura. Another school classifies the aura as following: the etheric field, the emotional or astral field, the mental field, the intuitional field, the spiritual field, the monadic field and finally the divine field. Another classification or a school classifies the aura as following: the auric field (the etheric field), the morphological field, the T- field, the L-field, the universal field and finally the geofields.

From these examples of classifications of the aura we can notice that most of the schools agree on a definitive and unarguable three fields which are: the etheric body, the mental body and the astral body. Beyond these three fields there are fields that are more complicated and arguable fields that participate also in an assistant role in the issue of the healthy human body and the aura as one wholeness of the physical human body and its auric fields or bodies since they are mixed and affect each other in different degrees.

Whenever we deal with the first three auric fields: the etheric field, the astral field and the mental field, we have something to do with the physical body because this category of auric field are relatively heavy and dense in their nature while the fields beyond the mental body are much lighter in density when we talk about the mass as vibrating energy.

When we examine the aura beyond the third auric field, the mental body, we deal with a spiritual and divine source of energy that are much lighter and less dense than the first three auric fields we have mentioned earlier. Even though each school is firmly believes in its beliefs and considers each auric field as a unique field regardless the fact that certain auric fields are more concerned with the healthy issues of the human body than other and that is essential in the treatment of the human body by methods that are falsely considered as mystical or ambiguous or even unproven.

If we take a look at those fields that are beyond the third field, the mental body, we should discuss the subject of the aura from a spiritual and divine perspective. The divine and spiritual like fields are existing in the auric field and they are important in the whole healthiness of the human beings but they are not in the same degree of importance as the first three fields concerning healthy issues of the human body as we will see later on.

There are different types of energy, thermal, electrical, magnetic, nuclear, kinetic energy etc. and that energy is only a different degree of the same thing which is the mass. In other word, the mass is the "figure" and the energy is its different types of faces.

The energy of the aura and specifically the etheric body is measurable. Although, the type of the energy of the whole aura is not an ordinary type of energy that the scientific men can define in obvious and definitive terms. One of the reasons is that we can not sense it with the help of our normal senses and our cognition can not realize it but despite that, the auric energy affects us positively or negatively in many ways that makes the aura subject an essential issue to understand at a satisfying level and that level depends upon the will of the seeker or the researcher to understand the nature of the aura's energy in a wanted level.

In some scientific sources the aura is described as a plasma field of energy that I do not agree with and in other sources it is described as an electromagnetic field which is near the truth of the reality and the nature of the aura. The most important thing that we should keep in mind is that this field is a biological one and it is not artificial. This means that the aura as a field is originated from our biological human body and it is linked to the outside of the human body to the whole universe. The aura receives its dose of vital energy through prana, the vital force, that is received from the whole cosmos and that nourishes every living organism on earth. We used to think that we are part of the whole universe, then we should by fact take in consideration that the human beings and the whole universe are one total unit. This unity should logically share many features and one of these features is the prana. This means that the universe that has made the humankind is not a dead universe. It is a living one.

We can notice here that the aura is always tightly linked with each biological process of the human physical body. We see that when we are starved for example, for one day or more, the glucose level decreases in the blood stream and that leads to the initiation of many enzymatic processes that in turn leads to the utilization of the fatty tissues that are stored in the body instead of glucose which is the usual molecule of energy production inside human body. We know by fact that the brain cells differ from other organs in the body in that it is entirely depending on the glucose in its nutrition when we are not starved and that can explain why some shamans is starving in purpose for one or few days in order to see the vision they need to see in their "traveling" to other worlds what they wish to see in order to be cured or to cure somebody else. The fatty tissues in the human body undergoes a catabolic process (catabolism means to break down to the original components) that makes the fatty acids, which is the result of the catabolism of fatty tissues, available in the blood stream which feed the neurons in the brain instead of glucose which is found in insufficient amount in the starving case.

From evolutionary point of view the human body during starvation is in a danger state and threatened not to survive, therefore the evolutionary mechanism of the human body must be in an alarm state and this enable him to coop better with the environmental challenges and we know that the chakra system that I will discuss later, which is one of the links between the physical human body and the aura of the human body is connected with the central nervous system that include the brain and its cranial nerves and the spinal cord and its spinal nerves.

The evolutionary mechanism of the human body is built in an adapted way and in this case of starvation, the neurons of the brain will function more effectively during the nourishment of the fatty acids molecules than the standard fuel which is the glucose molecules. So it is now easy to understand the mechanism that makes shamans more creative in their imaginations and more

sensitive to the outer signals. So it is not a supernatural phenomenon that does not have any medical explanation disregarding the fact that some people doesn't believe in those strategies that shamans, for example, use to enhance their abilities in order to cure themselves and others with their traditions that have been used for thousands of years for that purpose of healing.
Now we can explain the features of the first three fields of the human aura.

Etheric body

Etheric Body is the first field to discuss always because it is the nearest one to the skin of human body and because it is the densest field regarding the vibrating energy of its mass. It takes the form of the human body's surface and it is so powerful to keep the human organs and every biological particle in the human body healthy and isolated from the harmful environmental factors concerning the bad influences of other human auras and the bad influences of the environment of different types.

It is called sometimes the vital body because of its importance in keeping the physical human body healthy and intact. It is vibrating in and out of the human body in a harmonious way through the seven chakras of the human body that I will mention in some detail later on.

Astral Body

Astral body is a unique field because of its distinguishable colours. People who developed clairvoyance or are already clairvoyants has the ability to see colours of the astral body without any need of aid with any equipment. Each color represents a specific feeling in the human being and they change continuously depending on what the human being feels at a specific moment in time. It is less dense than etheric body and travel fast in the space and in higher frequency than the etheric body. Don't be confused with the "astral world" term because it is something else than astral body. Astral body is dependent upon our feelings, whenever we feel sad, envy, happy, enthusiastic, angry etc. this field or body of the aura changes accordingly. With "changing" I mean it changes its colour, intensity and shape continuously. The frequency of the vibrating energy of this field is characteristic for it. It is within certain interval of frequencies that belongs only to this field of vibrating coloured energy. As we can conclude here, the frequencies by which this field vibrates does not lie in the range of our normal vision of colours that we experience every day in life, therefore, as we said, it is only clairvoyant people who can see such colours.

Mental Body

Mental body is less dense than the etheric body, vibrating with a higher rate of frequency. Every thought that we think reflects itself in the mental body. Mainly, we think first and we feel later and in other minor cases we feel first and think later. This means that the mental body functions before the astral body in most of the cases.

Therefore, there is a correlated relationship between the astral body and the mental body and the telepathic phenomenon is concerned here in this field together with the astral body. Those who are gifted with telepathic ability can sense what other people think or feel through the changing in this field's characters and or the astral body's. Every thought has its characteristic form that exists in this field and beside that, the mental body changes its forms very quickly depending on the thinking activity of the person.

The activity of the brain regarding the thinking and the cognitional parts of the brain are concerned in the mental body while the emotional parts of the brain which are called the limbic system are concerned in the astral body. It is called the mental body because simply it is dealing with the pure mental cognitional activities of the brain like thinking function of the brain.

It is important to mention here that the aura with its different subtle bodies or fields are not arranged in layer like manner, i.e one above another on as many would imagine and as many pictures shows in many sources. In reality those fields are mixed with each other and they are in a constant movement and in a constant changing in their sizes, shapes and intensities.

The above mentioned features of the astral and mental bodies depend significantly on the individual's emotional and mental states respectively.

Now it is easy to imagine how these fields of energy change their locations, intensities, sizes and forms constantly.

PHYSIOLOGY, PATHOLOGY AND THE AURA

Whenever there is a study of the auric fields, knowledge in human physiology is very important. The reason for that close relationship between physiology and the auric fields is due to the very early manifestation of symptoms of the disease in the auric fields before the symptoms appear in the human physical body. Therefore a good understanding of human physiology is necessary to understand the defects in the auric fields of the human beings before it changes to pathological conditions as diseases.

Physiology is defined as the knowledge of the mechanism by which the healthy human body works normally and pathology is the knowledge of the disease initiation and progression in the human body.

There are many systems in the human body that works constantly and these are: the cardio vascular system, the nervous system, the endocrine system, the gastrointestinal system, the musculoskeletal system and the genital system.

These systems function normally if the functions of the organs that constitute these human body systems function normally. In the orthodox medicine, the initiation of the disease starts when there is an injured part of the tissue that belongs to a specific organ. Each system is consisting of organs, and when the injury occurs either by an internal or external factors the pathological process starts. External factors include for example microbes like bacteria and viruses and internal factors include a change in the function of certain cells like in the case of cancer or hypertension (high blood pressure).

To keep the normal function of the organs and tissues the individual should avoid unhealthy habits like smoking, alcohol, etc. and avoid as possible to be infected by microbes and keep a healthy habits like ,for example, eating a rich omega 3 fatty food, like fatty fishes to keep the cytoplasmic membrane (the envelop of the cell's contents) of the human cells and human tissues as healthy as possible and that would affect the aura positively by enhancing the function of the nervous tissues that constitute the entire nervous system. Unhealthy human tissue affects the human aura negatively. Those who smoke for example, have always a bad quality of the aura. The omega-3 fatty food has proven to make the cell membrane of neurons, brain cells, more flexible and that in turn lead to a better function of the neurons. The neurons transfer the electrical signals more rapidly which enhance the function of the brain and the spinal cord and their grove and fine nerve branches. The brain as a part of the nervous system has an important role in mental activity. Whenever the brain is sluggish in thinking, the aura that emanates from it is not active or strong enough as it would be in normal case. External causes of diseases are also a major threat to the human aura. A sick person has a "sick" aura. Microbes can cause tissue damage that disturbs the normal function of the tissue of the human organs which lead to a weak aura.

The endocrine system is defined as the group of ductless glands which secrete their hormones directly to the blood stream. The hormones distribute in the whole human body through the blood stream and these hormones affect their target cells by making the cells responding through cascades of internal cellular signals. The effect of the hormone is mediated according to the function of the hormone in concern.

One of the internal causes, i.e. the factors inside the human body that can cause a huge change in the character of the aura that permeates in all cases the inside and the outside of the human body, is the endocrine system. If the endocrine system is impaired, the aura becomes "fragile" and susceptible to the bad influences of other person's aura in the person's environment when such bad influence exists in some people as an example of external factors. Not only that but because the aura permeates each cell inside the human body, the human body becomes susceptible to microbes because of the impaired immunity and becomes easily exposed to other diseases and that in turn leads to a more deterioration of the human aura and the process take the shape of a destructive circle like pattern of deterioration in the human body.

The nervous system plays also a major role in the healthiness of the human aura. We know that each emotional, mental and physical activity is originated from the brain which is responsible for most of the instant changes of the aura's characters. The reason for that instant changing in the auras characters is due to the fact that the communication of neurons is electrical, compared to the chemical communication of the hormones, and its speed is higher than in the endocrine system, therefore it is normal that the changes in the aura becomes too much faster than in the changes that occur through the communication of the endocrine system.

Despite that direct influence of the nervous system on the aura, there is a usual and a well known pathway of the influence of the nervous system on the endocrine system and this pathway occurs through the nervous system itself. So we now see that the nervous system either influences the aura directly and it is the fastest way for result or through the endocrine system and that is the slower way of influence.

The effects of hormones on the aura are mediated by hormones of the endocrine glands that are secreted directly to the blood stream. These hormones reach their target cells, bind to their receptors in the cytoplasmic membrane of the cells, the envelope of the cells contents, and through a cascade of internal cellular signals the effects of the hormone is mediated. Through the RNA molecules (ribonucleic acid), the final result of this process is a protein molecule that has a certain function in the human body. The protein is either secreted from the cells interior side to the cells' surfaces or stay inside the cells to play a main role in the changes that occur to the human cells which are needed functionally and which were the purpose of the secretion of the hormone in concern.

All those processes in the endocrine system take time to occur and we can by such discussion conclude that the fastest way of changing in the aura's characters is by the nervous system rather than by endocrine system.

If our emotions or mental state change through the activities of our senses or thinking, the aura and especially the astral and mental body, that is concerned in the healthiness of the human physical body, change according to the change in the mental and emotional activity of the human body and through the chakra system and its nadis (we will explain nadis later on) that have a close relationship to the whole nervous system of the human body.

The human tissues consist of cells that are specialized to certain functions in different organs which make the biological organ systems of the whole human body. Each cell of the human tissue ultimately consists of atoms. Each atom consist of a nucleus and electrons that moving around the nucleus. The nucleus is charged with a positive charge due to the presence of protons that have positive charges while the electrons are charged with negative charges. Each electron generating its own magnetic filed due to the rotational movement around its own axis and due to the movement around the nucleus. Both movements are involved in the generating of the electron's magnetic field. The presence of the two poles of the atoms, the nucleus positive and the electron negative poles are responsible for the electrical field of the atom. Both the magnetic and the electrical filed composes the EM, the electromagnetic field, that is very important in keeping the integrity and healthiness of the human cells and the tissues.

If the EM field is altered for some reason, a sick tissue will ultimately be the result. The following is some of the factors that lead to the disturbance of the EM:

Natural Intrinsic factors like thunderstorms, cosmic rays, solar flares, gamma rays etc. and some artificial intrinsic factors like radiations from colour TV, radiations from microwave oven, aluminium vessels used in cooking and carbon monoxide fumes. Some intrinsic factors include: emotional stress, hormonal imbalances, infectious microbes and diet deficiency.

THE LINK BETWEEN THE HUMAN BODY AND THE AURA

The key factor here is the chakras. We mentioned the chakra system earlier but we did not discuss it in an enough depth that is needed to cover the aura issue. We can not think of the human aura without the chakra system because the chakras are the only parts of the aura that enable the aura to permeate the whole human body in a harmonious way. We can conclude that the aura without chakra system is unthinkable.

The chakras in reality are the places of the auric field that receive and emanate the fine type of energy, prana, that human body needs in order to function normally i.e. emotionally, spiritually and mentally. They are wheel like conical vortices that are part of the etheric body. On certain levels of the human body these conical vortices are located in pairs. Each single chakra is facing its mate and meets its mate at the tops of the conical shapes in the spinal column of the central nervous system.

Each chakra of the human body has its own characteristic colour and each chakra works optimally in the frequency range of the colour that belongs to the chakra in concern.

chakra   colour
crown   royal purple
ajna (brow)   indigo
throat   light blue
heart   green
solar   yellow
sacral   orange
base   red

It is important that you should avoid imagining that chakras' characteristic colours in the astral body of the aura are constricted to each region of the corresponding chakra. In fact, these colours can be every where in the aura and here we are talking about the astral body and not the whole auric fields since the colours of the auric fields refer mostly to the astral body.

We should notice that the table of chakra's colours is more concerned in the therapeutic effect of the normal coloured light that applied on chakras more than what each chakra emanates of its own coloured energy as light. So if we feed each chakra with its appropriate frequency of coloured energy (in the table), this will make the chakra absorbs its favorable and desired type of energy that makes the chakra healthier and makes it functions more correctly and in harmony with other chakras and with the universal source of energy, i.e. the prana that the chakra absorbs and utilizes during the whole life of the living human beings.

As we mentioned earlier we are part of this universe and our existence on earth is dependent on our environmental factors such as air, water, food and the essential source of vital force, the prana. The chakras are the locations where the prana or the universal energy are received and distributed throughout the whole body through what is called the nadis. The Nadis are channels or pathways that run throughout the whole human physical body and which facilitate the distribution of prana to every part of the human physical body.

There are about 72000 nadis in the human body but the main two are pingala and Ida in Indian traditions. Each one is located at each side of the body and they cross each other at different levels in the human body. The third major nadis is called sushumna which does not cross the body's halves.

We know that the energy of each chakra of the etheric body rotates in its standard and normal frequency in healthy human body. If the frequency of rotation is increased or decreased than the normal level, then the chakra is in a state of imbalance and the chakra is either in hyper- or in hypofunction and needs to be adjusted through the aid of many cleaning methods.

Sometimes the flow of energy from the cosmic sources ,the prana, which is here called (the primary source of energy), becomes blocked at the entrance to the chakra or it becomes blocked at it way to the nadis from the nervous system. Here the prana is called (the secondary source of energy). In both cases the chakra becomes sick and will not function normally.

There are seven major chakras in the human body and many other minor chakras. The seven major chakras are: crown chakra which is located at the top of head, third eye or ajna chakra which is located at the level of the forehead, throat chakra which is located at the level of the throat, heart chakra which is located at the middle of the chest, solar plexus chakra which is located at the navel level of the body, sacral chakra which is located at the sacral level of the vertebral column and root chakra which is located at the end of the vertebral column.

The crown chakra is unique because it has a connection with the divine source of energy in the cosmos.

These chakras take the shape of funnels that radiate the prana, the universal biological energy or sometimes it is called the (vital force), to the cosmos and at the same time they receive the prana from the outside of the human body i.e. the cosmos.

The chakra can be blocked partially or totally by some factors like anxiety, trauma or sudden psychological shocks which make the chakra sluggish and the energy inside it rotates in a slower or higher rate than normal. In this situation, the harmonious energetic connection with other chakra nearby will be disturbed and this will participate in the abnormal function of the aura and predispose the human body ultimately to pathological diseases.

The main and the long lasting effect of the aura on the human body occurs through the endocrine system of the human body. The human body's pineal gland which receives its nourishment of the auric fields through the part of the aura at the level of the top of head where the crown chakra is located. A healthy pineal gland reflects its healthy function on the crown chakra that in turn reflects itself on the auric field at the level of the top of the head.

Now we can give a summarized ide about the function of each

endocrine gland and its hormones in order to understand the importance of the endocrine system for the auric fields and the importance of the auric fields to the endocrine system.

The pineal gland has an organized cyclic variation of the secretion of **melatonin hormone** during 24 hours of time. This hormone controls the sleep pattern of human beings. Melatonin is synthesized from the neurotransmitter serotonin of which tryptophane is the precursor. An important fact to remember here is that melatonin decreases and increases periodically in a rhythmic pattern. Melatonin synthesis is inhibited by light and stimulated by darkness. Melatonin function in the human body is to induce sleep and to inhibit puberty. This rhythmic cycle of sleep and wakening is mediated by light signals from retina of the eye and from the thalamus, hippocampus and pineal gland itself. The oscillatory cycles of impulses to pineal gland are coming from suprachiasmatic nucleus (SCN) that is situated in hypothalamus region of the brain.

The pineal gland that in some scientific sources is said to be a residue of the evolved man and it does not have any function is by fact a false statement.

When we speak about the master gland in the human body, we always mean the pituitary gland (hypophysis) for the reason not of its size but because of its multifunction that this gland has on other glands in the human body.

The pituitary gland is the most major gland in the human body. It consists of two parts, the anterior lobe (frontal lobe) and the posterior lobe (back lobe). It lies in a bony walled cavity called sella turcica in the sphenoid bone at the base of the skull and it is operated through the third eye chakra.

The posterior lobe secretes **antidiuretic hormone (ADH)** and **oxytocin hormones.**

ADH hormone is one of the most important hormones in keeping the osmolality and the volume of the body fluids in the normal level. Osmolality and water "concentration" are two faces of the same coin. Normal ADH level keeps the excreted urine in normal compositions of water and salts. Excessive ADH due to the abnormal function of the pituitary gland leads to an excessive amount of water in the urine, in other words, the human body excrete large abnormal amount of diluted urine. A decrease in the secretion of ADH leads to the excretion of small amount of concentrated urine. In both cases, the extra cellular fluid, the fluid that lies between cells, and the cells themselves, become either hyperosmotic or hyposmotic compared to the plasma normal osmolality. (Plasma is the blood without the blood cells).

Stimulation of the region of female breast during sucking of the baby activates the posterior part of the pituitary gland to secrete **oxytocin hormone** into the bloodstream as a reflex.

Now we list the hormones of the anterior lobe of the pituitary gland which are essential hormones. The anterior lobe of the pituitary gland secretes the following hormones:

Growth hormone (GH)

Thyroid stimulating hormone (TSH)

Adrenocorticotropic hormone (ACTH)

Luteinizing hormone (LH)

Follicle- stimulating hormone (FSH)

Growth hormone (GH) or somatotropic hormone (STH) constitute 5-15 mg of the pituitary gland and it is stored in very huge amount in the pituitary gland. GH is secreted at 2-hours intervals. A peak in GH secretion occurs about 2 hours after a deep sleep which is during the stage 3 or 4 of sleeping waves.

GH decreases the uptake of glucose by the muscles and instead increases the uptake of amino acids, the building parts of protein and increase protein synthesis in the muscles. GH also increases the synthesis of protein and increases the number and the size of cell in the bone, heart, muscles and chondrocytes (cartilage cells). GH has its positive effect on all types of tissues in the human body. In adipose tissue it increases lipolysis, degradation of fatty tissues, is one of the examples.

Thyroid stimulating hormone (TSH) is another hormone that pituitary gland secretes to the bloodstream. TSH stimulates the release of thyroid hormones which are released from the thyroid gland.

Adrenocorticotropic hormone (ACTH) is another hormone secreted by the frontal lobe of the pituitary gland. Pituitary gland is a master gland because of the factors we mentioned earlier and also because of the many hormones it releases to the blood stream. Therefore as we said it has a main control on other glands in the human body.

ACTH binds to receptors on adrenal gland cortex. Adrenal cortex cells produce in turn **cortisol and aldosterone hormones**.

The function of aldosterone hormone is simple. This hormone reuptakes sodium in kidneys before sodium joins the urine, therefore any abnormal increase in aldosterone hormone lead to a hypertension (increased blood pressure).

We can perhaps recognize the word cortisol because it is almost the same as the word cortisone which is a suppressor for immune system, anti-inflammatory and antiallergic.

Cortisol hormone decreases the protein stores in the extrahepatic tissues (hepatic means liver related) , increase blood glucose concentration by inhibiting utilization of glucose in peripheral tissues, in other word, cortisol has antiinsulin effect in tissues like muscular tissue and adipose tissue (adipose tissue means tissue where the cells contain fat) and decreases the uptake of glucose for energy. During fasting cortisol allows epinephrine and growth hormone to catabolize (break down) adipose tissue.

Thyroid hormones are secreted from the thyroid gland are important for the growth and development of the human body. It increases all cellular metabolic activity in all tissues of the human body. The thyroid hormone increases the use of food for energy. The growth rate of young individuals is increased. The mental activity is stimulated and the activities of all other endocrine glands are increased.

Thyroid hormones (TH) increase the number of the mitochondria.

Mitochondria is the factory where the energy molecules ATP (adenosine tri phosphate) are produced in the human body.

TH manifestations are obvious on growing children. Those who have deficiency of TH show a delay in growth. Also TH promote the growth and development of the brain during fetal life and during the first years of postnatal life.

The thyroid and its nearby parathyroid gland are operated through the throat chakra.

Parathyroid gland secretes **parathyroid hormone (PTH)** from four glands which are located behind the thyroid gland.

PTH regulates the plasma level of calcium. Plasma can be defined as the blood without blood cells. We should mention here that thyroid gland affects calcium level in the blood by secreting calcitonin hormone (CT).

The thymus gland is operated by heart chakra. In thymus gland a T lymphocyte (one type of the cells of the immune system) undergoes a modification so that T lymphocyte can binds to different antigens (foreign sites on the microbes). This process occurs few months before and after birth so a defected heart chakra after this period of time does not affect the thymus gland too much.

The adrenal and pancreas glands are operated by the solar plexus chakra. The endocrine part of the pancreas is the islets of Langerhans that secrete **insulin hormone** to the blood stream from beta cells. Insulin mediates the transport of glucose (the usual energy molecule that release energy) to the cells of the body. Without insulin, the body's cells starve and a diabetes type I becomes manifested. Alpha cells in Langerhans cells secretes glucagon hormone which also has many function in the metabolism of the human body.

The spleen is operated by spleen chakra, the spleen chakra is not always mentioned in the human chakra system but it exists if we look at the system in detail. The spleen function is to fight the infection in the human body and act as a reservoir for the fluid of the human body.

Ovaries and testes are operated by sacral chakra. The whole glandular system is operated by the root chakra. The testes are responsible for producing sperms and ovaries are responsible for producing ovum.

If we take a close look at all those functions of the endocrine glands, we begin to think seriously about the auric fields and its effect on endocrine glands and the effect of the endocrine hormones on the auric fields.

By nourishment of the human cells, tissues and organs we mean that the vital energy of cosmos, the prana, which is everywhere in the universe and everywhere in our living biological human bodies is running through every cell, tissue and organ. Whenever there is an enough and a circulating prana, the human body is alive otherwise it is only a piece of mass without a core of vital energy that usually operates in a harmonious way with the whole biological system of the human body.

Through the direct effect of the aura on the human tissues, the aura is nourishing the organs, tissues and cells with the vital energy that tissues need to keep its vitality and to function normally.

Chine's medicine through acupuncture is a try to "guide" the energy of the first layer of the aura, the etheric body, through needles and focus that energy to the area of the body that has deficiency in the etheric body.

Every part of the tissues vibrates in harmonious frequencies with the frequencies of the human aura. Every part in the whole universe vibrates in its own frequency and the aura and the human body is normally part of the universe as a whole system of energy flow that vibrates continuously.

The human body receives its nutritional dose of vital force, the prana, through the aura itself. That stream of vital energy circulates through the body via chakra system to nourish every cell in the human body.

Nadis which are the channels that transmits the prana, from the chakra to the whole human body is the key factor or the link between the chakra and the nervous system with its ganglia, plexi and the endocrine glands. Therefore, the nadis determine the nature and the characters of the nervous system with all its branching from the brain and the spinal cord. The focal and important point that attach the chakra to the spinal column is called bindu and it is essential part of the auric field that should be intact.

If the transmission of the vital force or the prana is blocked through this system of subtle energy, the physiological status of the human body becomes imbalanced and if it persists, it could lead to acute or chronic diseases in the human body due to improper nourishment of prana for the human cells and tissues.

The nervous system is divided into two parts, the voluntary and involuntary nervous system. The subdivisions of the involuntary system is sympathetic and parasympathetic systems. (we will discuss the nervous system in part 5). The main effect of the vital force that flows through nadis are observed to be mostly on the sympathetic and parasympathetic system of the human body while the voluntary system functions in a less dependent mechanism on the auric fields and the vital force.

Finally, we should mention that nadis, nervous system and endocrine system are the three major factors that play a huge role in the integrity of the human body as a whole functional unit of the auric fields and the physical human body.

THE HEALTHY HUMAN BODY AND THE HEALTHY AURA

Each healthy biological system is dependent upon other healthy systems that work together in the same physical and functional unit which is in this case, the human body.

Whenever there is a contamination of some kind in any biological system of the human body there is symptoms of the disease and there is a cure. Concerning the auric fields the damages or symptoms if we can call them are invisible to our naked eyes but they exist defenatively. If such damages persist, they would manifest themselves as clinical symptoms of pathological diseases, i.e. the symptoms appear in the physical human body.

The human tissues are totally depended on the human aura in order to continue being alive and function normally.

Without a healthy aura the healthy tissue becomes a sick tissue and with a complete absence or defected aura, which in normal case permeates each part of the human cells, the cells will ultimately die.

Many people that have the ability to heal other persons utilize their own auric fields and therefore their aura becomes depleted of its potential energy. The healthy aura is important in keeping the individual alive and the individual can in rare cases die in the extreme situations of depleted potential energy of the aura as he becomes weaker in time.

Those who used the universal source of auric energy for healing purposes do not lose the potential energy of their own aura. Animals and plants have also their own aura concerning the etheric body in specific. Plants are enveloped and permeated by their own etheric body that keeps the plants alive. We see that for example when shamans used pieces of plants in treating or cleaning their clients they don't used those plants again because these plants have lost their healthy etheric auric field since they gave their energy that is kept in the aura in the process of cleaning the individual in concern.

If we have a depleted etheric body it is a good ide to find an alive tree and put our backs facing its trunk in order to make an exchanging of energies of human's and the tree's aura that help the individual to fill his aura with healthy energy from the tree.

From evolutionary point of view the earth we used to live on has its own magnetic field that has dominated the evolution of human beings through a long period of time, therefore, it is normally that the aura and the etheric body in specific is composed of a magnetic field as one of its component beside the electrical field that takes a larger space of discussion that it is not concerned in this book.

One known tradition of healing the human body is by a magnet that man can buy from stores and put one pole, the south or the north on the ill places of the human body either to stimulate or to inhibit the magnetic part of the human aura for that part of the human body which is ill. The north pole of a magnet used to have an excitatory effect while the south pole used to have a calming effect.

Colour therapy is also a known way of healing. By color therapy we mean that different colours of light are applied to different part of

the human body to heal it.
The colored light is a vibrational wave of energy that we daily often ignore because of the absence of knowledge in this branch of science. Each chakra colour has its unique frequency of vibrational waves that is in harmony with the vibration of each chakra of the human body. The chakras can absorb the positive and nourishing energy of the coloured light waves to supply each chakra with the vital energy. That type of vibrating energy can be absorbed in turn to the human aura and specifically to the etheric body and astral body which are an important link between the human body and all other fields of the human aura.
The healthy astral auric field has bright colours rather than dark muddy colours that dominate the defected and the leaky aura where in this situation, the aura instead to repel the negative type of energies from the outside of the human body, it absorbs the unfavorable types of energies that the human body comes in contact with.

The brighter the colours of the astral auric field (astral body), the healthier the aura is. The most balanced and ideal healthy state of the aura is manifested itself in pure white colour which is the composition of all perfect healthy colours together. Those people who have very balanced chakra system and very healthy chakras, their aura appear like a pure white coulors and every one that is in nearby these masters feels himself calm, worm and happy. Again, the most predominant colour's manifestation occurs in astral body where the clairvoyant people can see those colours normally without any external aid like auric photography. Those people are gifted and they are very few in the population.

Vigorous, fast moving and shape changing waves of the aura emanated from very healthy persons are a typical case. Those people are very immune from the outside "attack" of the bad influence of other person's aura if such bad contents existed nearby the auric field of the typical healthy persons. The healthy people have always bright colours in the astral auric field reflecting the healthiness of the biological system of the human body. A depressed person, a low self esteem persons or sick persons usually have weak auric fields and that is concerning all the fields or bodies of the aura we mentioned earlier. Their auric fields are susceptible for all types of hazardous factors outside the human body. Those people possess relatively depressed immune systems that make them easily infected by microbes or fungus and usually have prolonged time of recovery from an infection or an inflammatory process compared to healthier persons that have healthier aura.

We can completely understand here the close correlation between the auric fields and the healthy status of the human body. In fact they are in a reciprocal relationship, i.e. they affect each other like an endless direction of a circle.

When the human body becomes sick or injured for some reason, the auric fields becomes also defected. The astral colours become cloudy and more black colour becomes incorporated in the astral colours of the auric fields which make it looks like dirty muds which indicate the unhealthiness of the auric field.

The pathogens (the microbes) that initiate the disease process is an important factor in weakening the auric field of human body. The pathogen initiates the inflammatory process which is the feature of almost all diseases in the human body. In another word each pathogen is associated with an inflammatory process unless the microbe has an incubation period. The inflammation that is characterized by swelling, heat, pain and redness is a disturbing factor for the flow of the energy in the nadis of the chakra system and that leads in turn to a blockage in the flow of prana, the universal biological energy, in the human body. This leads also to gaps in the auric fields which become unhealthy and weak. The process of the inflammation can be externally on the surface of the body or internally in different organs and tissues of the human body. Another interesting phenomenon of the auric fields is the collective unconsciousness. Every one of us lives together with the family members, among his or her friends, in a city, a community or in a whole land. In each of these cases there is an influence of the unconsciousness of other people on the person's own unconsciousness who naturally belongs to the group of people in concern and that is called collective unconsciousness. So, if an ethnic group, for example, live among a bigger group of people who have a hatred feelings for that minor ethnic group or for a person who belongs to that ethnic group then all the persons in the bigger group will affect the minor group or the person that belongs to the minor group by the total unconsciousness of the bigger group in a negative and destructive way which is mediated by the auric fields. If someone hate, loves, depressed, happy, envy or loves others, etc., the person's emotions and feelings are always and constantly reflecting themselves in the atmosphere of the auric fields and they are potentiated in effect when there are more people nearby, who share the same feelings and emotions. We all sometimes have noticed that we feel strangely uneasy and that there is something "wrong" in ourselves when we, for the first time, meet some group of people we don't know. This is because of the difference in the emotional and mental features that exist between the person and the group of people in concern.

Because the collective unconsciousness is of emotional origin, this phenomenon is mediated by the astral body that we discussed before. The psychologist, Carl Gustav Jung, mentioned this phenomenon in his writings and believed that it has an effect on the unconsciousness of the person. The more the likeness of the features of thinking and or feeling that reflects itself in the auric fields of the group, the more is the effect on the person via his own auric fields.

The person receives the collective unconsciousness through the chakra system which is, as we said, part of the auric field and the transmission of informative feelings of the group is like a porous sponge that fills its holes with the collective unconsciousness and squeezes the contents of itself to the unconsciousness of the minority.

But here we can notice that the person is also a part of the group and it is illogically to isolate him from the group unless the group's content are a lot of persons like in the case of a country, a city or even a school. The majority of people that live in these places used to share the same characteristic features mentally and or emotionally because of the "group effect" that has a psychological explanation which is not concerned in this book.

The collective unconsciousness becomes none collective if the majority does not share the same feelings or mental pictures that the persons inside the group used to have in order to make the collective unconsciousness alive and effective.

The early treatment of a defected aura during its early stages of deterioration has always a better prognosis than the late treatment when the defected area of the aura has already damaged parts of the human physical body.

THE NERVOUS SYSTEM AND THE AURA

Every evolved organism on earth has a nervous system and has the
ability to use it in order to survive many hostile and threatening
environment that the organism faces daily in life. Human nervous
system is so advanced and is capable of facing the hostile
environment with a unique way that differentiates him from other
organisms.

I preferred to put the nervous system in a separated chapter because
of its importance in the auric fields and also because of the
complexity of its contents.

If we take a look at the human nervous system we can find that it
can be divided into two parts, the structural and the functional
nervous system. The structural nervous system is usually divided into
two parts, the central and the peripheral nervous system.

The central nervous system is subdivided in turn into the spinal
column and the brain while the peripheral nervous system is

consisting of the spinal nerves that are originated from the spinal column and the cranial nerves that are originated from the brain.

The functional nervous system is a little bit more complicated than the structural one and it can be divided into the voluntary and the involuntary nervous system.

It is called voluntary because we as human beings have full control over its final results as motoric activities while in the case of the involuntary nervous system, we do not have any control over its function.

While the voluntary nervous system consists of many nerve branches that are motoric, the sensory branches receive the signals via our senses.

By sensory branches of the nervous system we mean all the nerve fibers that transmit the senses' signals from the outside of the human body to the brain cortex therefore it belongs to the involuntary part of the nervous system while the motoric branches transmit the movement's electrical signals from the cerebral (brain) cortex to the voluntary striated muscles of the human body. We should here also mention an important type of functional divisions of the involuntary nervous system which are the sympathetic and parasympathetic parts. I am going to explain the sympathetic and parasympathetic nervous system in some detail later on but let us now take a look at the functional unit of the whole nervous system which is called the neuron, the specialized cell of the nervous tissue. The neuron consists of a cell body which is called the soma and a tail like structure which is called the axon. Sometime the axon is surrounded by an interrupted sheath which is called the myelin sheath and the interruption points are called nodes of Ranvier. The purpose of this sheath and Ranvier nodes are to facilitate the transmission of electrical signal through the axon to make the electrical signals move faster. The transmission of information through the axon which is the longest part of the neuron occurs through electrical impulses. The most important electrical charged ions here which are involved in the transmission are calcium and sodium ions. We can notice that the outside of the cell membrane of the neuron is charged likewise the inside of the neuron and they have opposite charges. With the movement of the charged ions through the neuron's cell membrane, the electrical charge of the inside and outside of the cell membrane changes and according to that change the action potential is initiated. The term action potential is used here to indicate that an electrical impulse has been originated or transmitted.

Now the reader may stop reading, wondering and asking himself or herself: "But why should I know all that?"

The only thing I can say at this moment is that these facts are necessary in order to get a closer picture of the auric fields that has a reciprocal effect on the different functions of the human's organ systems. Despite that the reciprocal relationship between the nervous system and the auric fields, the nervous system affect the auric fields much more than the auric fields affect the nervous system except in rare cases such as those who have telepathic abilities.

We have now two components to discuss, the tissue of the nervous system and the tissue other than the nervous system. The first one is mostly electrical in nature while the second is "neutral". The neutral tissue does not mean that it does not have an emanated type of energy. As we said before, every piece of mass like a tissue or a piece of iron or an old chair, all radiating very low and fine level of electromagnetic field that is very characteristic for the item in concern. So in other words the tissue even if it is a dead one, radiating a certain level of electromagnetic frequencies. But we are dealing with a living tissue and that means that there is a prana, the cosmic and the vital force of energy that permeates only the living tissues. Besides that, the auric fields permeate each part of the living tissue of the human body.

If we take a look at the subtle energy of the nervous system we can find that there is a difference between the nervous system and the living normal none nervous tissue. The nervous tissue has its own electromagnetic field that is much more powerful than the non-nervous tissue. And that powerful field enables us to look at the function of the heart muscle with the help of electrocardiogram (ECG) or with the help of electroencephalogram (EEG) when we examine the brain's activity. It is well known that the heart has well organized nerve branches that innervate the heart muscle with a rhythmic pattern of electrical impulses so it is not surprising to know that the heart muscle has a highly electrical activity.

As each negatively charged electron rotates around its own axis and around the nucleus, a magnetic field is generated as a result of that rotation. We remember that the nucleus of the atom is positively charged and that lead to the generation of the electrical field. Both electrical and magnetic field participate for the biological electromagnetic field that is found in the normal tissues of the human body.

Now if we ask ourselves, what is the relationship between that EM field and the aura? The answer for this question is quite rational than scientific. As people evolved since ages on our planet, these two fields has become mixed with each other and the final result is a dominant auric fields because it is more powerful than EM field of the human tissues (except in the case of the electromagnetic field of the nervous system that is found in the heart and the brain).

We should mention here that the electromagnetic field of the auric fields is not identical concerning the quality factor with the electromagnetic field of the heart or the brain. The auric fields are relatively more magnetic than electric when it is compared with the electromagnetic fields of the brain and the heart as long as their functions depend on electrical current in millivolts. In auric fields the electrical current that is transmitted everywhere in the human body and around it is actually much less than few millivolts. We can summarize that the human aura has more magnetic component than the electromagnetic field of the heart and the brain while it has relatively less electrical component than the electromagnetic field of the heart and the brain.

The sympathetic part of the nervous system with its sympathetic ganglia and parasympathetic part of the nervous system with its pre and post ganglionic nerve fibers are an important component of the nervous system concerning the auric fields.

The sympathetic and parasympathetic nerves innervate the organs in the human body that function involuntary like the heart, the stomach, the kidneys, the small and large intestine, etc.

Such organs that are innervated by both sympathetic and parasympathetic nerve fibers are working without our control, therefore, they function automatically depending on the need of the organ of stimulating or inhibiting stimuli to function in a harmonious way in each organ system of the human body.

We know that the voluntary innervation of those parts of the body like the skeletal muscles are much stronger regarding the will of man than the autonomic (involuntary) innervations therefore the auric fields has stronger effect on the autonomic nervous system than the voluntary nervous system. Only a delicate changing in the auric fields of the human body makes a remarkable changing in the function of the organs of the autonomic nervous system.

The brain, cerebellum, has an interesting region which is called the limbic system. The limbic system is the part of the brain that is responsible for feelings, emotions and memory. It consists of few parts: amygdala, cingulate gyrus, hippocampus and septal nuclei. Some or all of these regions are activated under emotional stress and how we feel in different situations. The astral body of the auric fields is a specialized field where emotions and feelings are manifested as we mentioned before. The relationship between the limbic system and the astral body is little ambiguous and vague.

As we know every cause has its effect and this is one of the natural laws of the existence we are living in.

When we consider the limbic system as a cause, the astral body will be the effect and vice versa. Every time there is an activation of the limbic system the reflection is found in changing the shape and colours of the astral body of the auric field. And in the same way, every time the astral body changes its forms and colours, the limbic system is the most sensitive part in the body to that change in the astral body of the auric fields.

As we said before, the flow of prana is through the chakras into the inside of the human body and from the human body via chakras to the outside of the human body.

We can notice that this process occurs at the level of the ajna or the brow chakra and by the logical and rational thinking, the effect of this change will be only at the level of the auric fields that is at the same level of the ajna chakra. Well, the truth is not. Because the astral body change its form constantly and very quickly, ajna chakra's colour which is violet can be seen in other region beside the ajna chakra where the level of the limbic system is located. In this way we can assure you that there is no firmly and unique relationship between the colour of each chakra and the position of the endocrine gland or any system or organ in the human body. By this generalization we do not exclude the fact that the effect of the reciprocal influence of the auric fields and the somatic (physical) body at the characteristic levels of the chakra system occurs more intensively at these levels than other locations in the human body.